Sweary Nurse
Coloring Book

Get FREE printable coloring pages and discounted book prices sent straight to your inbox every week!

Sign up today at:

www.adultcoloringworld.net

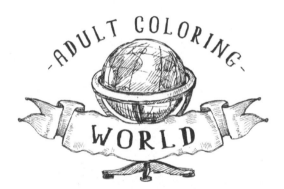

I'M THE
FIRST PERSON
YOU SEE
AFTER YOU
SAY "HOLD
MY BEER AND
WATCH THIS
SHIT"

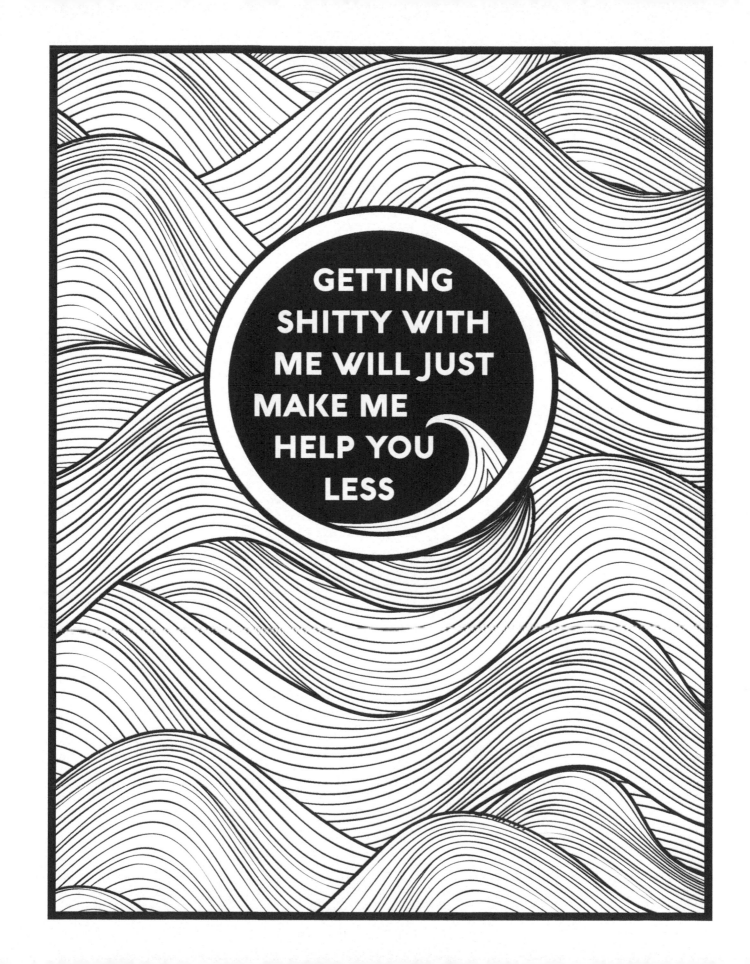

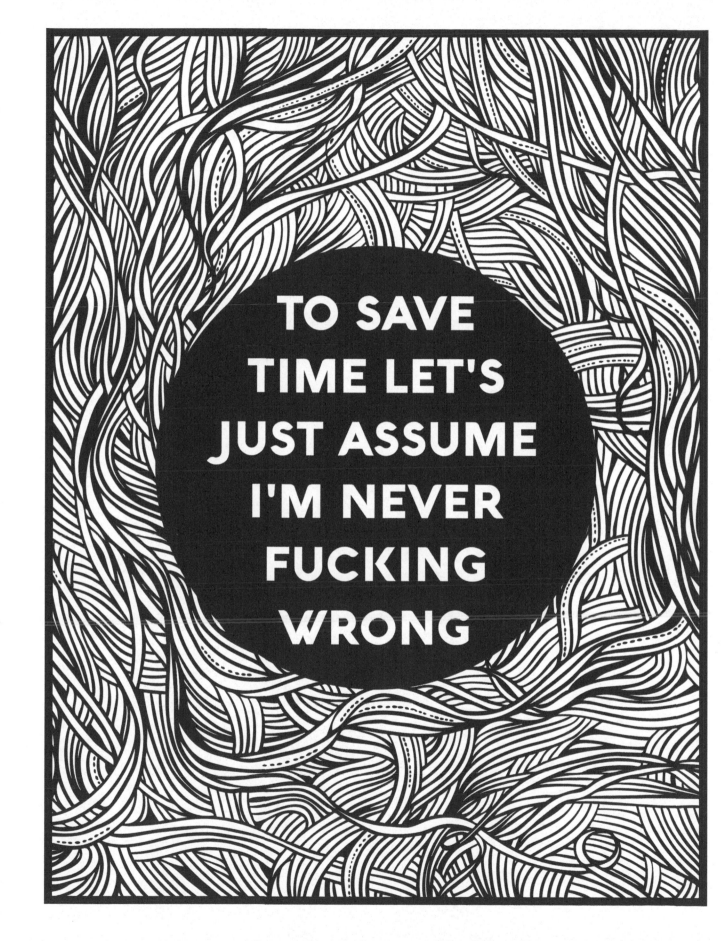

I'M A NURSE BECAUSE EVEN DICK HEAD DOCTORS NEED HEROES

I DON'T CUSS
LIKE A SAILOR.
I CUSS LIKE A
FUCKING NURSE.

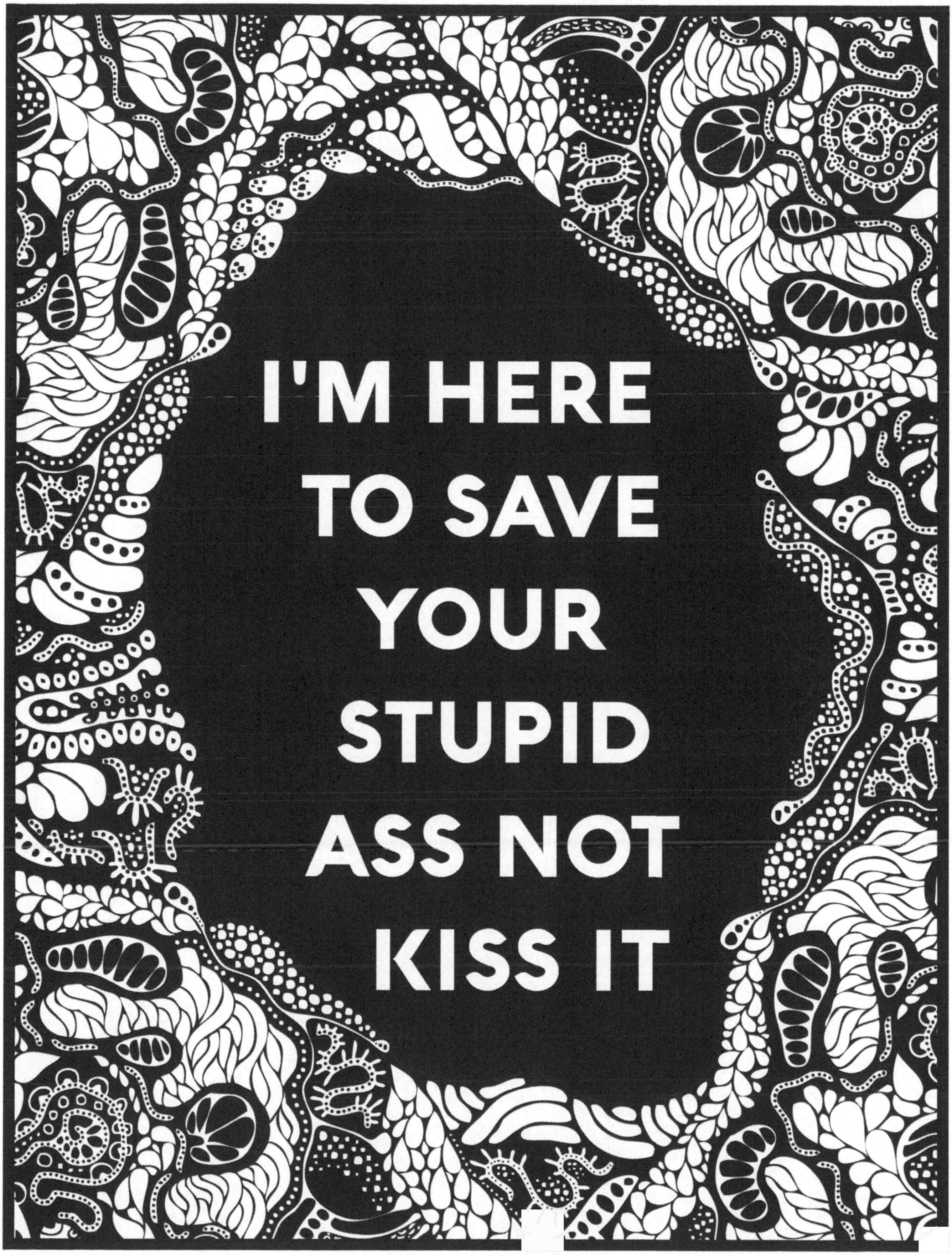
I'M HERE
TO SAVE
YOUR
STUPID
ASS NOT
KISS IT

I HATE BEING
SO FUCKING SEXY
BUT I'M A NURSE
I CAN'T HELP IT

I'M PRETTY
MUCH HERE TO
STOP THIS TWAT OF
A DOCTOR FROM
KILLING YOU

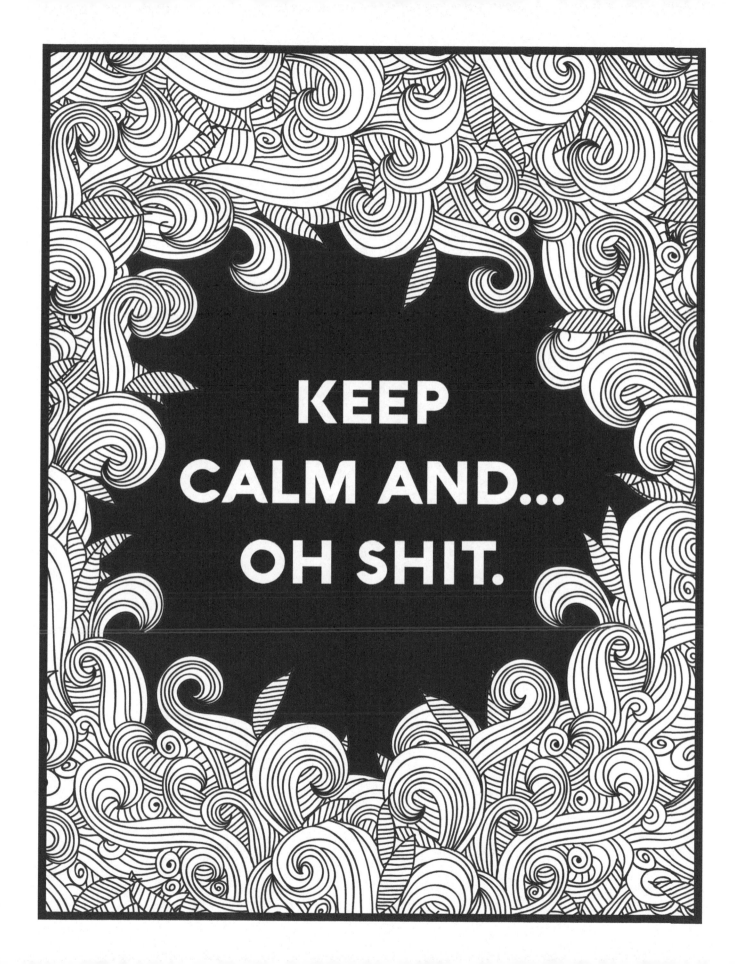

A DOCTORS
HANDWRITING
DECODER WOULD
BE FUCKING GREAT
RIGHT NOW

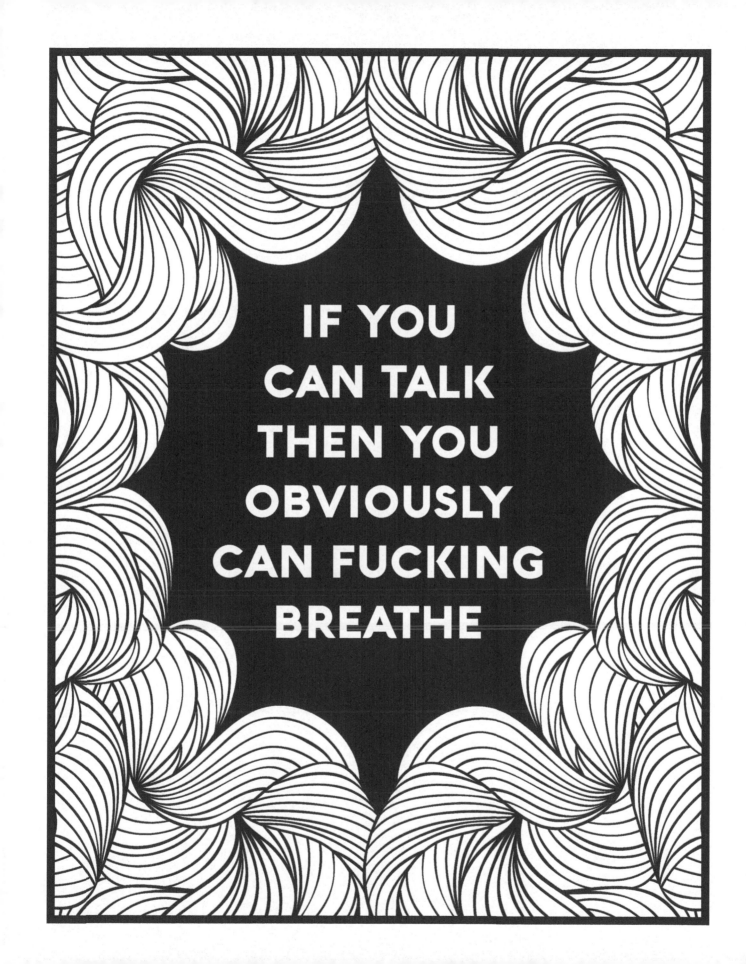

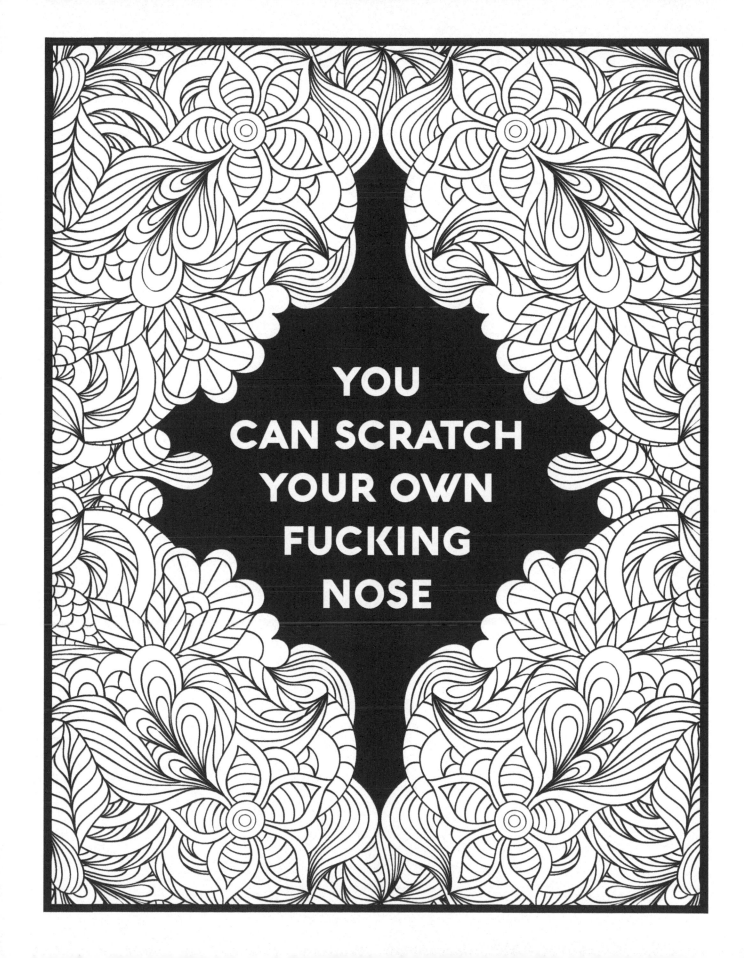

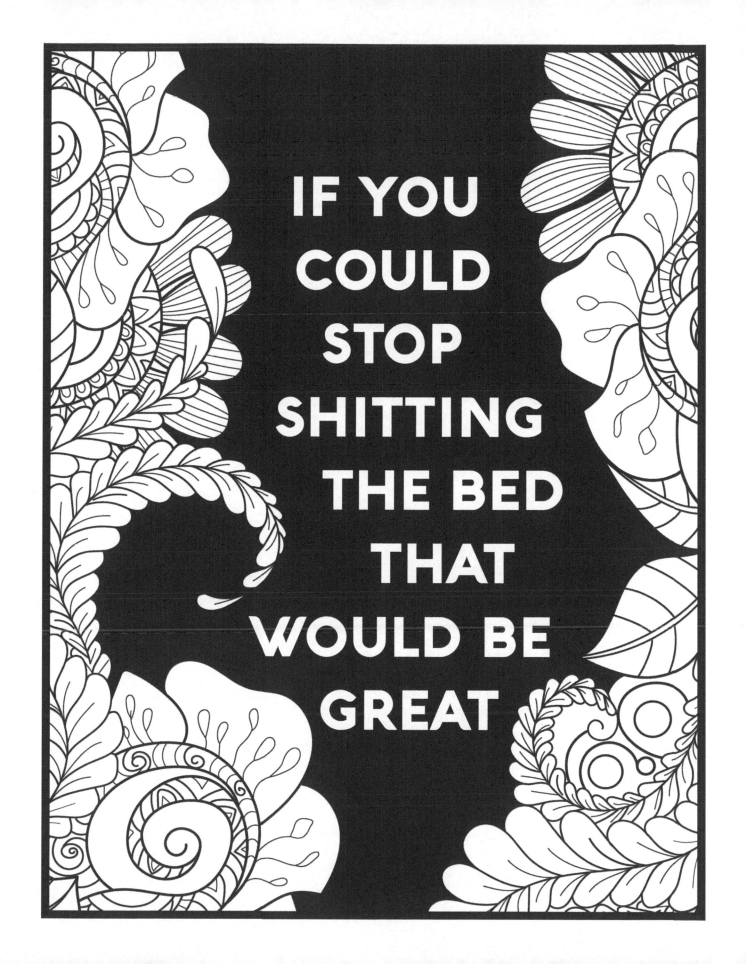

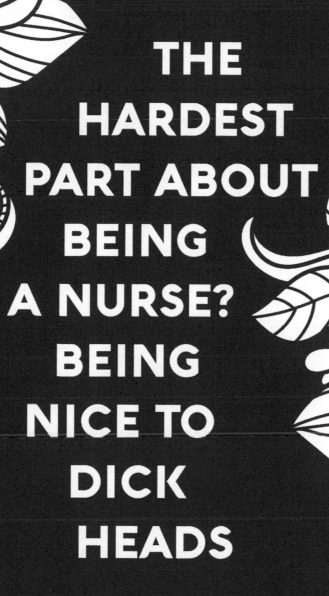

THE HARDEST PART ABOUT BEING A NURSE? BEING NICE TO DICK HEADS

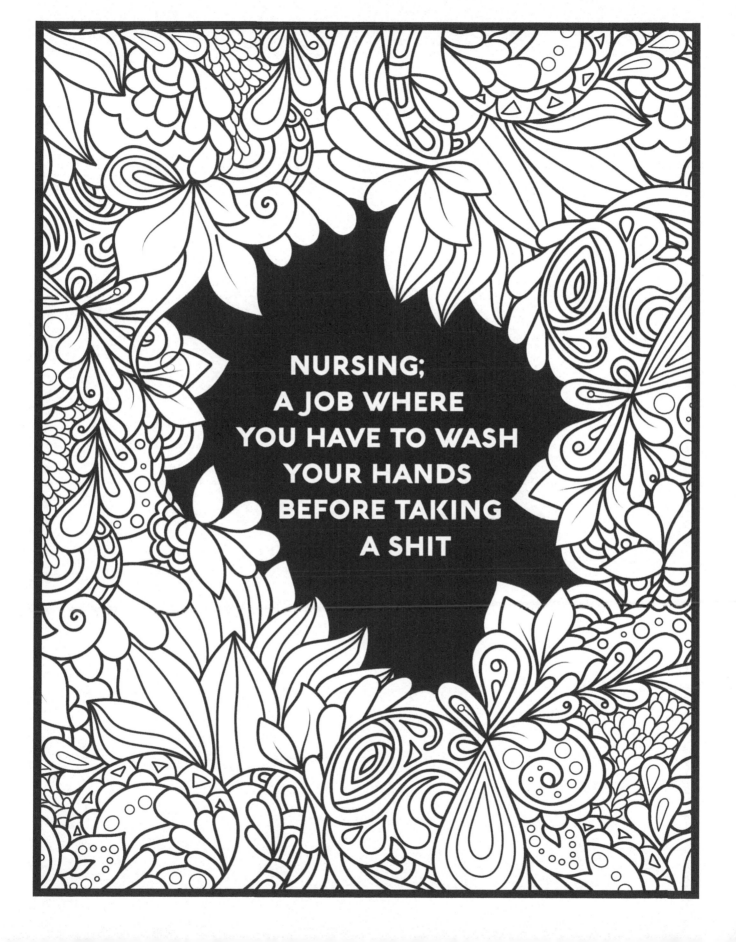

THE CLOSEST
I'VE GOT TO WATCHING
A FILM THIS YEAR IS
SEEING FIFTY SHADES
OF SHIT

IT TOOK ME
TEN MINUTES
TO GET YOUR
WATER BECAUSE
SOME POOR
FUCKER IS
DYING

TELL ME MORE ABOUT HOW YOUR PAIN IS TEN OUT OF FUCKING TEN

I SHOULDN'T HAVE TO TELL HUMANS TO NOT EAT THEIR OWN SHIT

THE PAIN IN
YOUR HAND IS FROM
HITTING THE FUCKING
CALL BUTTON FIFTY
TIMES AN HOUR

I SILENTLY MOUTH "WHAT THE FUCK" AT LEAST TEN TIMES EVERY SHIFT

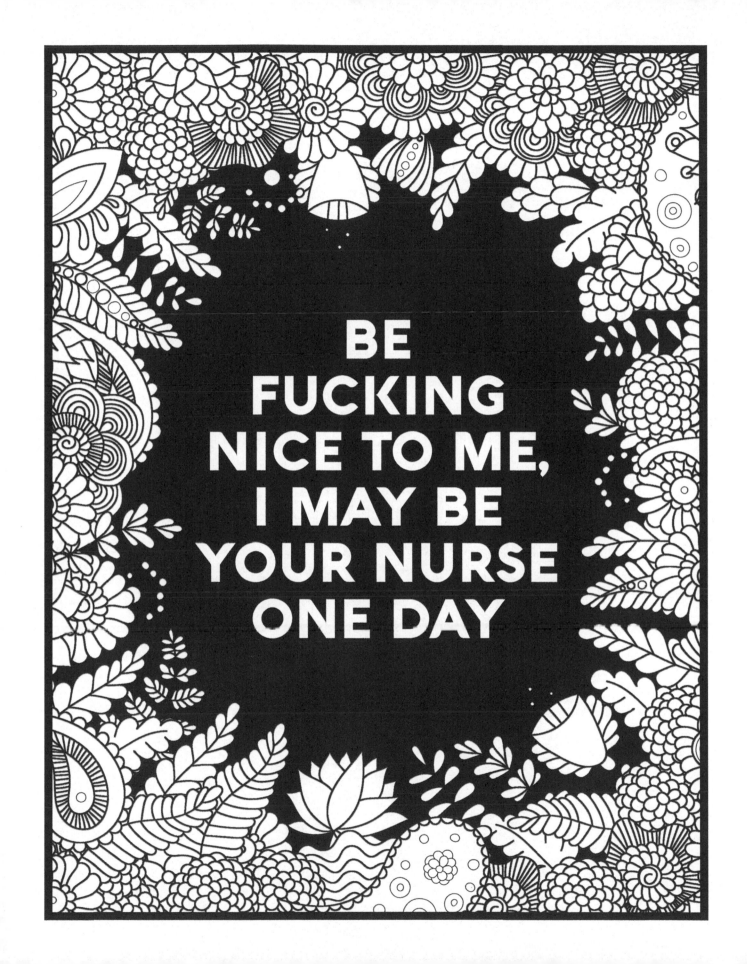

NURSE? NURSE? NURSE? NURSE? SOUND FUCKING FAMILIAR?

LUNCH BREAK?
BATHROOM BREAK?
AIN'T NOBODY GOT
TIME FOR THAT
SHIT

THE BIG H ON THIS BUILDING DOESN'T STAND FOR FUCKING "HILTON"

I SEE YOU

HAVE A SEVERE

CASE OF FUCKING

PRETENDINITIS

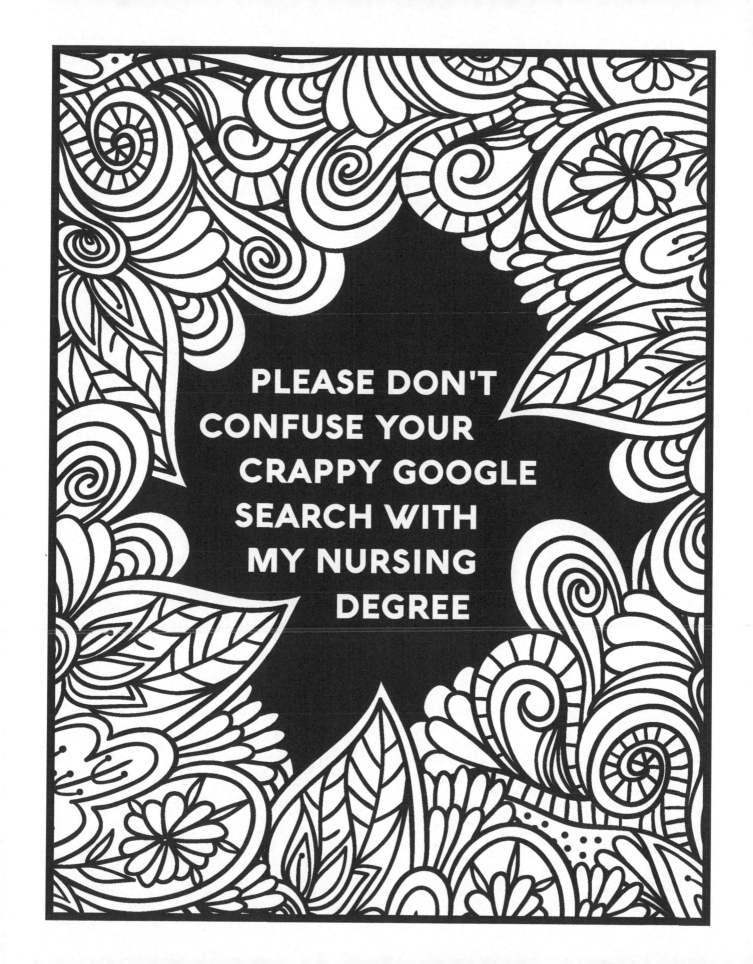

NURSING; WHEN YOU'RE NOT SURE IF IT'S TUESDAY OR FUCKING SATURDAY

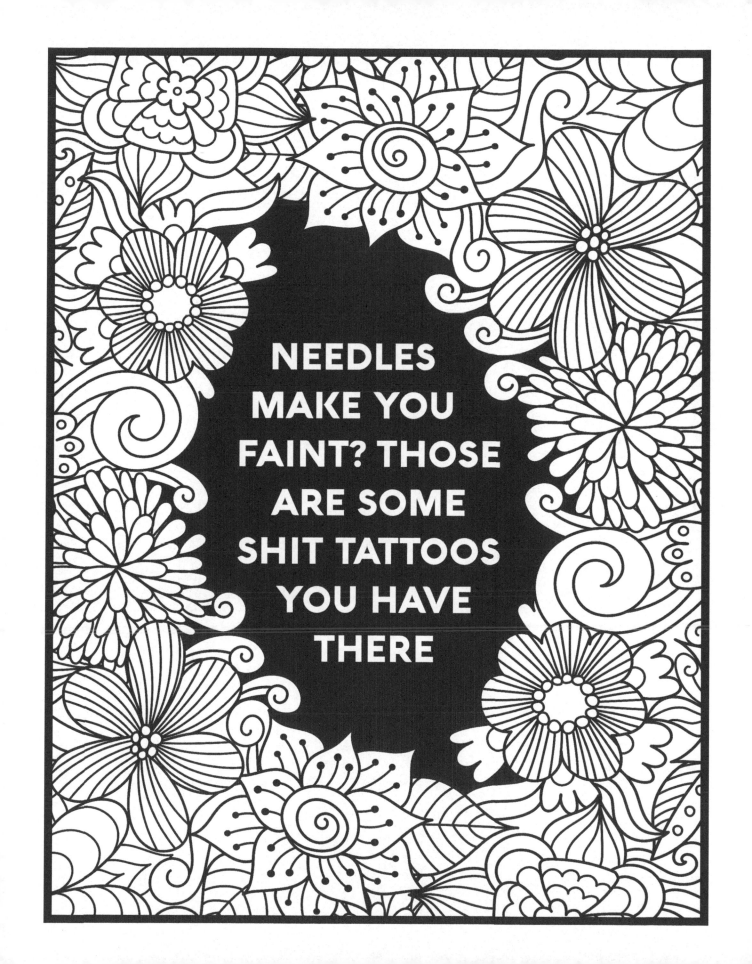

REALIZING YOU'LL TOUCH ANY OLD SHIT AS LONG AS YOU HAVE GLOVES ON

WHEN AN
INCONTINENT
PATIENT GETS PUT ON
A FUCKING DIURETIC.
THEN YOU KNOW
URINE TROUBLE

BE A NURSE THEY SAID. IT'LL BE FUN THEY SAID. TWATS.

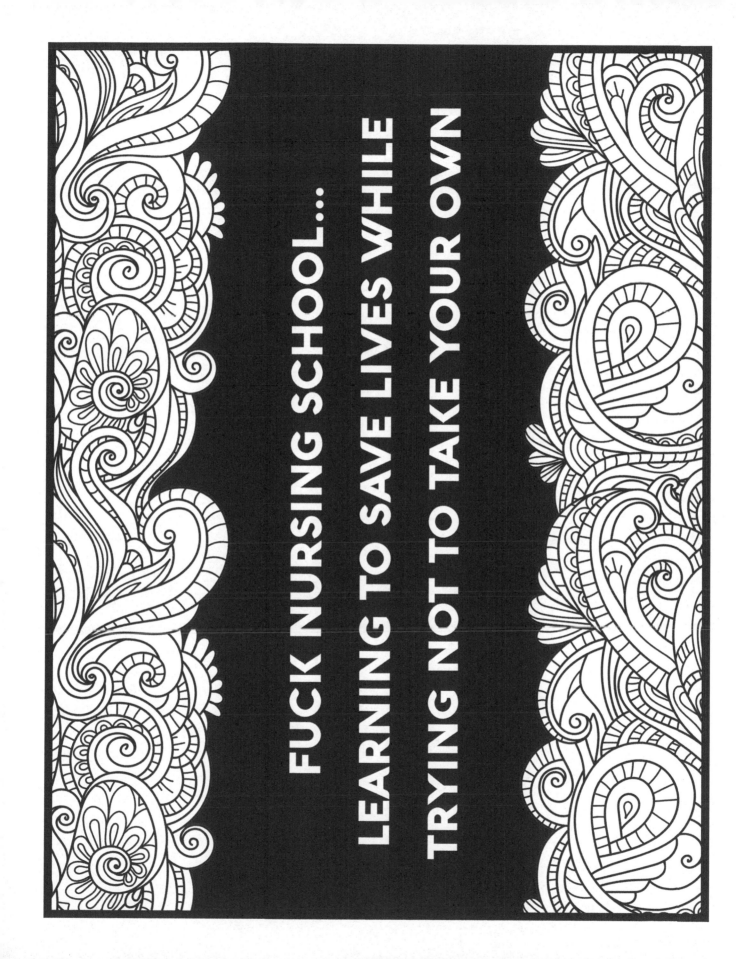

I NEVER THOUGHT I WOULD GIVE SO MUCH OF A SHIT ABOUT NICE VEINS

YOU
CAN'T FIX
DICK HEAD
DISORDER
BUT YOU
CAN SEDATE
IT

I'VE SEEN
MORE COCKS
AND VAGINAS
THAN MOST
HOOKERS

A PICTURE
OF A NURSE
SITTING DOWN?
CLEARLY
FUCKING
PHOTOSHOPPED
THEN

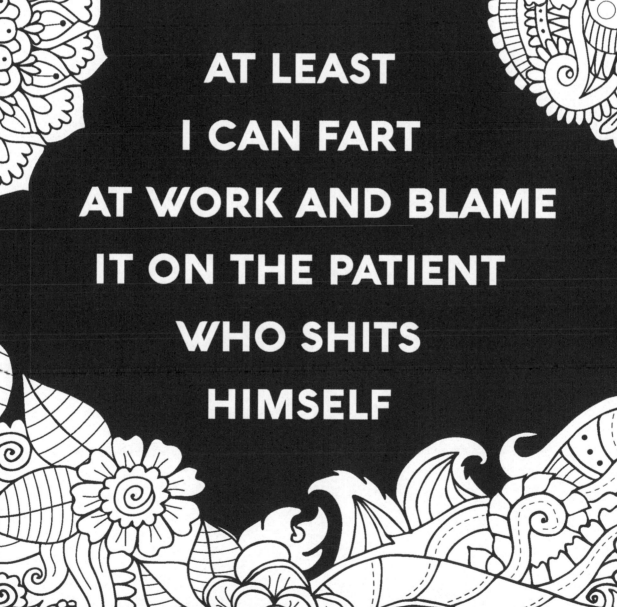

AT LEAST
I CAN FART
AT WORK AND BLAME
IT ON THE PATIENT
WHO SHITS
HIMSELF

IF YOU
HAVE MY PEN,
I WILL FIND
YOU, AND I
WILL FUCKING
KILL YOU

WRIST
RESTRAINTS,
BECAUSE
SOME THINGS
ARE WORTH THE
SHITTING
PAPERWORK

COLOR TEST PAGE

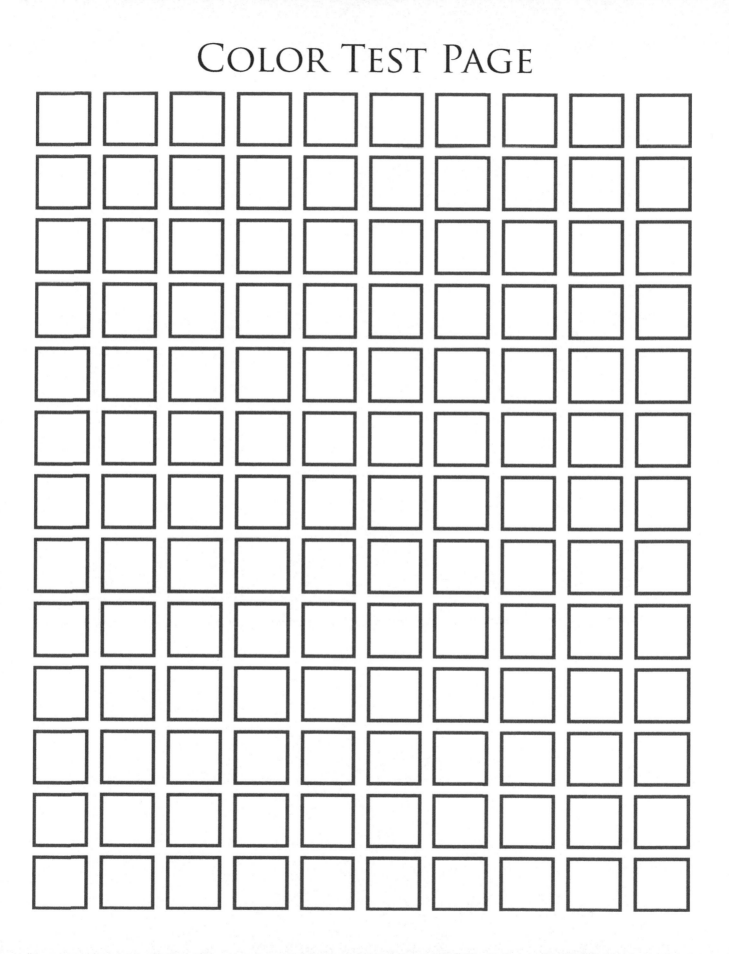

COLOR TEST PAGE

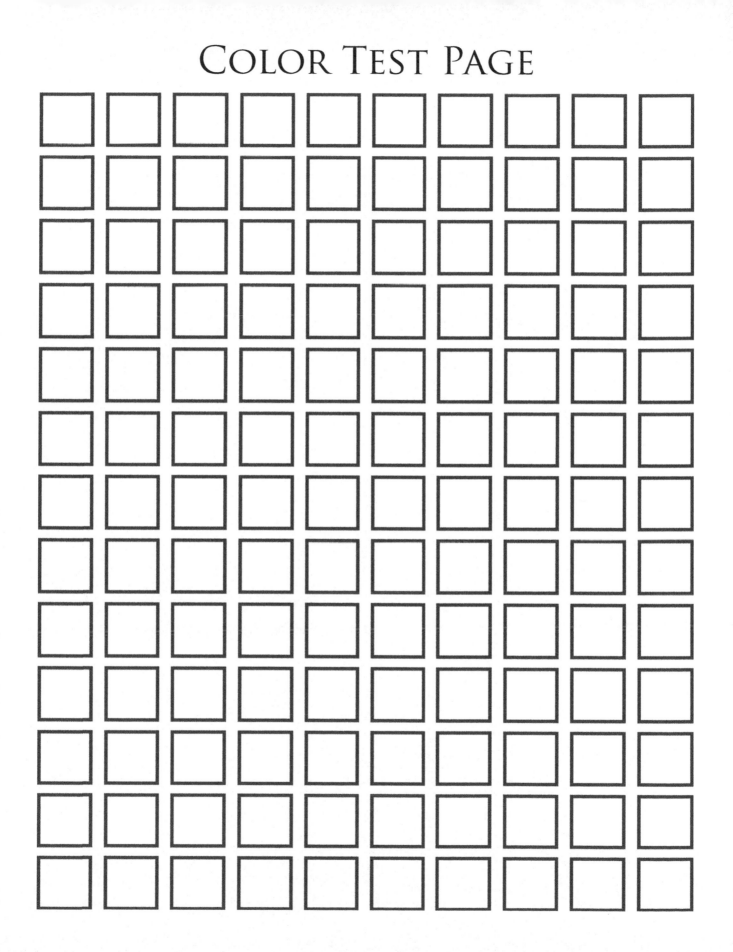

Made in the USA
Middletown, DE
30 April 2022